PICTURE YOURSELF , DO IT NOW !

Infinite Weight Control BAA

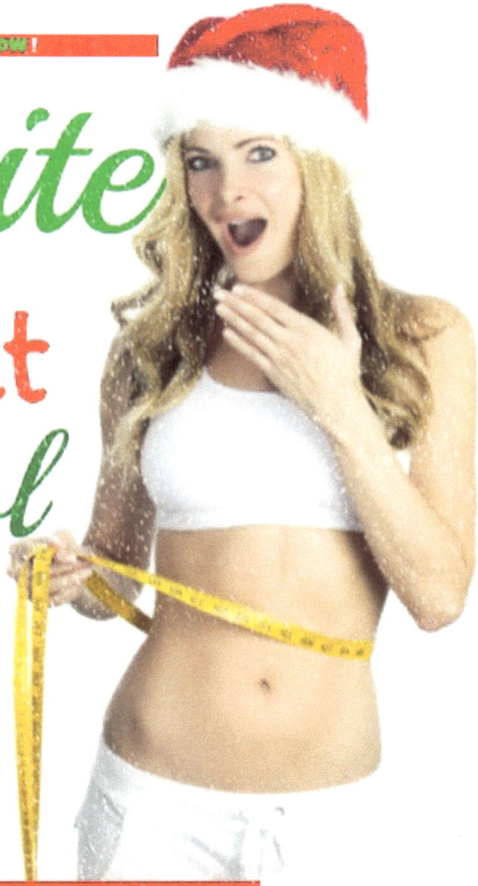

Lisa Kristinardottir

BEFORE, DURING AND AFTER HOLIDAYS WEIGHT CONTROL !

INFINITE
Weight Control
BAA

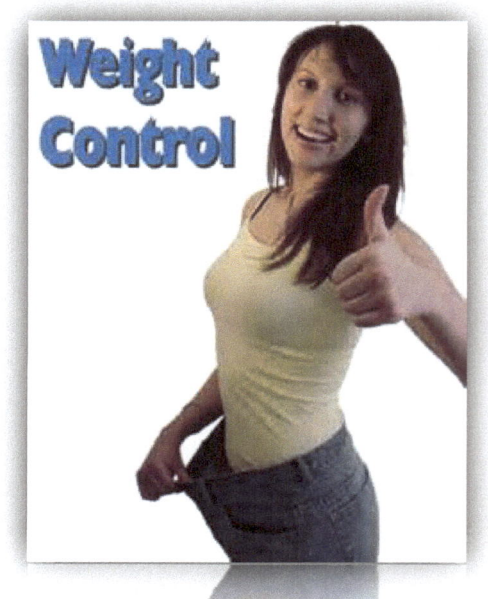

Lisa Kristinardottir

Lisa Kristinardottir

Infinite Weight Control BAA

ISBN-10: 1505387620

ISBN-13: 978-1505387629

Lisa Kristinardottir

DEDICATION

To my beautiful and most-loving family ARAM
(coded first-letters, each of your names, ha!)

…and my dear dear great friends, helpers and angels in

Russia, Iceland, Greenland, Scandinavia, USA, Europe,
Australia, Asia, Japan, Korea, Vietnam, China, Africa,
Middle East, Hawaii (yes, I haven't forgot about you, no
way!), Canada, Mexico, Argentina…

and…

angels all over the world where I may not be able to thank
you enough for your kindness, generosity and love! It is
not to be forgotten to me in this life or any other.

I could NOT have written, edited
and published this small book without YOU!

May your lives be happy always
now and forever!

Takk Takk (Thank You) Bless!

Lisa Kristinardottir

CONTENTS

Lisa Kristinardottir

ACKNOWLEDGMENTS

This book contains material protected under International and U.S.A. and International Federal Copyright Laws and Treaties. Any unauthorized reprint or use of this material is prohibited.

No part of this book may be reproduced or transmitted in any form or by any means, electronic or mechanical, including photocopying, recording, or by any information storage and retrieval system without express written permission from the author / editor / publisher.

NOTES TO YOU MY DEAR READER

While the author (me ;-) of this book have made reasonable efforts to ensure the accuracy and timeliness of the information contained herein, the author and publisher assume no liability with respect to loss or damage caused, or alleged to be caused, by any reliance on any information contained herein and disclaim any and all warranties, expressed or implied, as to the accuracy or reliability of said information.

The author makes no representations or warranties with respect to the accuracy or completeness of the contents of this work and specifically disclaim all warranties.

The advice and strategies contained herein may not be suitable for every situation. Please take care to check and double-check facts every time! I have been very diligent in keeping my writing factual, to-the=point and useful for me and you! Enjoy AND benefit!

It is the complete responsibility of the reader to ensure they are adhering to all local, regional and national laws.

This publication is designed to provide accurate and authoritative information in regard to the subject matter covered.

BLESS YOU ALWAYS

YOU ARE

THE MOST BEAUTIFUL

PERSON

EACH AND EVERY DAY

OF YOUR PRECIOUS LIFE

HUGS & KISSES

LIS

1 INTRODUCTION

PICTURE YOURSELF SUPER NICE!

DO IT NOW AND MORE IMPORTANTLY...

AFTER THE HOLIDAYS AND BEYOND!

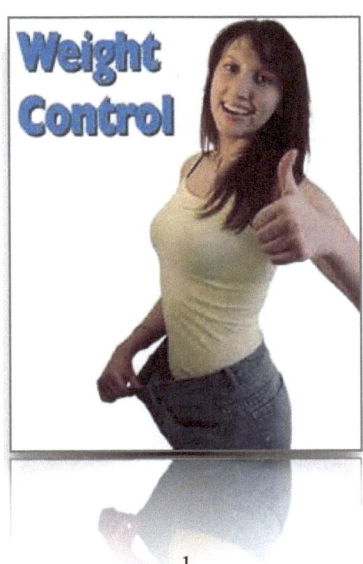

This book is all about **WEIGHT CONTROL** *during* the holidays and *immediately* after.

Any holiday. Pick any one out of so many great festive ones you enjoy with your loved ones!

In this day and age, having a diet or weight control plan is absolutely essential, yet many people don't have one.

The question on everyone's mind is *"if I get a weight control plan, how do I commit to it with such a busy lifestyle?"* The simple answer is, create a weight control plan around your busy life schedule. In this article, I'm going to reveal to you how to put together a simple plan that caters specifically to your needs.

Not surprisingly, most people **DON'T** have a weight control plan. Reasons include lack of time, no motivation or just bad experiences with weight loss fads that produced no results.

To get the best results and stay committed, read through **ALL** the chapters in this book and you will *defiantly* AND *definitely* *achieve* the best of results possible. Yes, it's in the mind! and… the body CANNOT live without the mind!

Thanks so much for your time in reading my piece on this subject.

2 CONTROL NOW!

Controlling Your Weight During The Holidays.

**Should NOT be a strenuous activity,
NOT mentally NOR
physically!**

READ MORE

TO

MAKE SURE!

FOR

EVER!

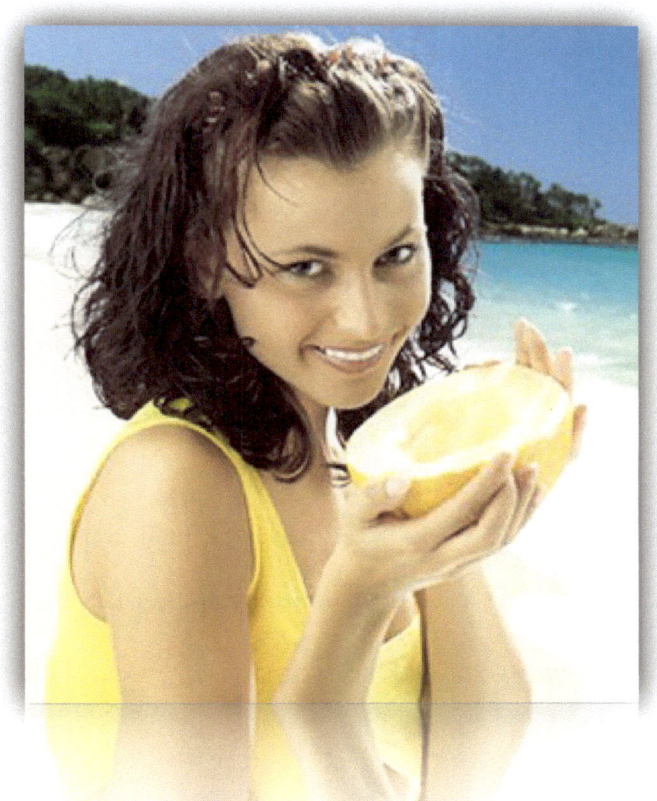

You ARE the most beautiful. NEVER forget that!

Weight watching is **NOT** a conscious process when you're on

your toes for months together. But when the holidays set in,

your weight **IS** on you alone.

Controlling your weight during the rushing holidays isn't a tough job. Just as you make plans for your family and yourself for enjoyment, include health as a member too.

Weight control is possible through the dedicated effort of an hour and making the rest of the day fun and abuzz with activity. Holidays leave you with more time to take care of your body and skin, and bring the weight under control without much distraction. That also means *excuses*. Don't give into them, ever again. Be very conscious of this at all times…

Managing weight issues shouldn't be anything like the robotic monotonous exercise program it is made out to be. You can involve your family and friends to lighten up the weight loss regime.

You don't really need to draw up determination reserves to watch your weight go down; only get yourself mobile when you'd rather give in to the temptation of squeezing in inactivity to take rest.

Be Regular In Your Habits

Holidays are meant for you to stay out late without an alarm to force you up before the sun rises up too. But don't make it your temporary way of life so you find it difficult to effortlessly slip back into your work routine.

Sleep *on time* so you give your body and mind sufficient time to rest and digest.

Don't oversleep or lie in bed an extra hour if you don't need to. Eat your meals on time. In fact, use the absence of rigid working hours to tailor your eating habits to the healthiest.

House Jobs

There's always something to do in the house. Plan in advance what you want to clean up, wash and throw and do it yourself. Keeping busy doesn't allow for much weight gain and you'll be surprised at how much domestic exercise can be got out of putting your home in order, like you'd want to do with your fitness levels.

Doing your own laundry, using the vacuum cleaner, cooking your meals and dusting and cleaning the house keeps you active and makes good use of the food you eat to provide energy.

Move Around, Hey c'mon! Get going...

If there's a technological appliance meant for your convenience, remember it has been invented to replace your own effort and energy spent.

Bypass the help and do your jobs on your own. It's much better for you!

You cannot find a good enough substitute for the TV or Internet show watching, playing games or some other www-related activity…but remember, you can skip the elevator for the stairs if your health allows you to.

Walk to near blocks instead of driving and stretch or spot-jog while watching the TV. Walk around while on the phone and keep your things in high places so you stretch to reach for them.

Eat Healthy, please.

It's VERY important!

Undoubtedly, you cannot avoid the parties and get-together which comes with lots of delectable but fattening food, but you can limit them and stick to your food chart.

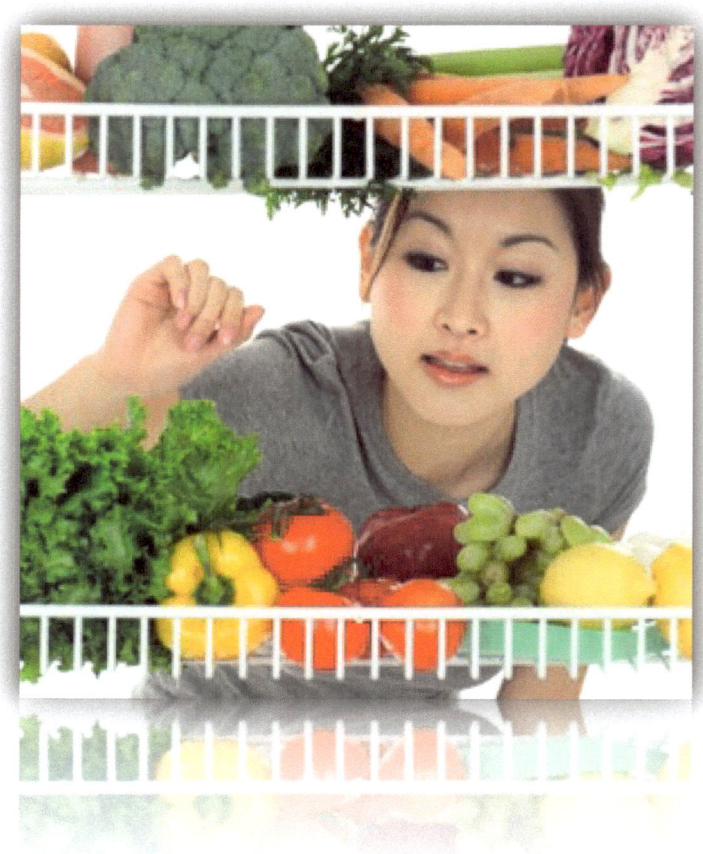

Avoid oily food and shop for fresh green vegetables and fruits in season. Eat smaller and frequent portions in a day comprising of uncooked vegetables and salad. Include fruit bowls in between meals when you feel hungry. Cut down on starchy food like boiled corn and refined bread or rice.

When you go someplace for a visit, stick to uncooked food for the most part and eat smaller portions.

Don't drink too much at night, especially, as the liver is overworked and the alcohol is then deposited as fat in the body. This adds to the visceral fat which is dangerous for your organs. Drink adequate water to help the digestion. Drink a full glass before going to bed and one immediately after waking up.

Hit the Gym

During the holidays, you have a lot of *extra time* on your hands which can be suitably divided into relaxation, enjoyment, chores and personal care. For people with long working hours, going to the gym drains them further and is thus avoided so they can pay attention to the household and the family.

Health neglect is further deepened with the presence of young children who need parental attention and care. Month-long holidays are the best time to foster your health and focus on controlling your weight without the guilt factor figuring in if you have children. Go to the gym thrice a week and enlist a personal trainer to give you detailed assistance in your workout.

Lose the Boredom

If the gym comes close to a jailed exercise routine from which you have no escape, then you can explore other options which you can go for with your friends too. Dancing classes are held everywhere, and allow anyone to join regardless of age.

You can sign up for one with an interested friend and it is a good idea to go with someone who also seeks to keep the weight under control. If everyone else is on vacation abroad and you find yourself battling your eating urges alone, then motivate yourself by joining classes for a trained dance form.

You'll keep yourself busy at home too, practicing to master the moves. Join an aerobics class for a full work out. It doesn't leave you very tired and pumps in the energy and tunes your body into shape.

You have greater flexibility of timings during the holidays, and so registered classes don't have to interfere with the holiday schedules you have in mind.

Don't Compromise On Exercise

Exercising doesn't entail hard to move equipment in all cases. Go for a walk or better still, run a few laps around the neighborhood park in the mornings. If you don't have the facility, wake up early and jog along your block. Skip at home with proper shoes on and supplement it with floor exercises. Stretch to warm your muscles up before any intense exercise.

Every holiday season brings with it the promise of wonderful memories and possible new experiences you'll munch on for life. But whatever the obligation, either at work, or catching up with family during the holidays, health is never secondary. Controlling your weight has numerous benefits and long breaks can be very well utilized to realize the goal.

3 HOW TO LOSE "HOLIDAY" WEIGHT GAIN

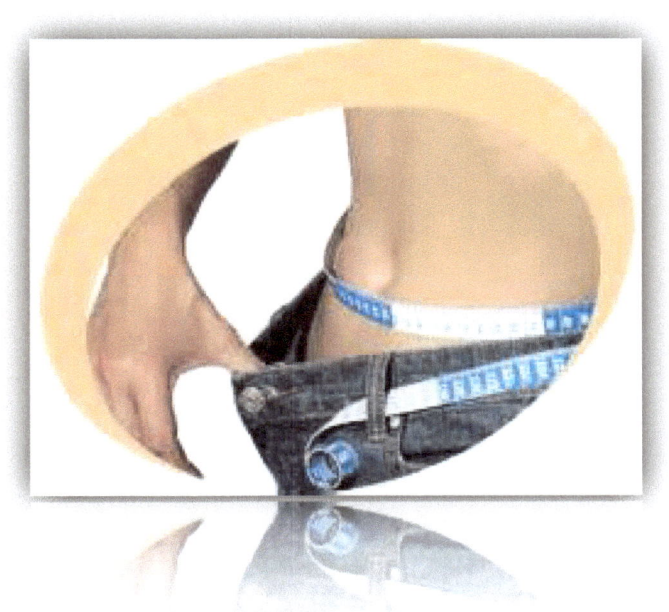

Holidays make for joyous opportunities that inspire many people to overeat, which often is the best part of occasions like Thanksgiving, Christmas and the Fourth of July. You pay the price, though, when you step on the scale and realize you've gained weight, or worse, you try to put on your favorite jeans and they don't fit. To keep weight gain from escalating, indulge your appetite during the holidays, but have a plan of action in place to shed the pounds as soon as you resume your normal everyday routine. Discuss any weight loss or exercise concerns with your health-care provider.

1...2...3...4. Ready?

HINT, HINT...

.... - > GO TO

...........................THE NEXT PAGE

...........................PLEASE!

PRACTICAL STEPS:

Go!

Step one

Reduce your calorie intake. On the first day after the holiday, put any sweet and fattening treats in the freezer for another time, or simply throw them out. If you normally eat fatty and sugary foods, reduce your sugar intake quickly by drinking water and tea instead of soda and fruit juice. Immediately after the holidays, replace candy, bagged snacks and desserts with fresh fruits and vegetables, lean meats, low-fat dairy products and whole grains.

Step two

Keep track of everything you eat and review your food journal daily. Write down your food intake in a notebook or use your smart device to keep video and audio journals of what you eat. Being aware of what you eat can serve as an effective reminder of which foods to avoid as you work on dropping holiday pounds.

Step three

Increase your daily exercise. After the holidays, resume your normal gym routine if you have a membership or join a nearby gym. If your local gym is cost-prohibitive, take one or several walks daily. Walking doesn't impact your budget and you may gain the added benefit of relaxation by walking in the park, at a lake or around a shopping mall. Depending on your current weight and how fast you walk, you could burn between 60 and 360 calories per day.

Step four

Join a support group. A support group can help you stay on track if you have difficulty letting go of certain holiday foods or need motivation to exercise on a daily basis. Employers, churches and community centers often offer post-holiday weight-loss support groups to inspire wellness practices before and after an indulgent break.

4 WEIGHT LOSS, NO GAIN!

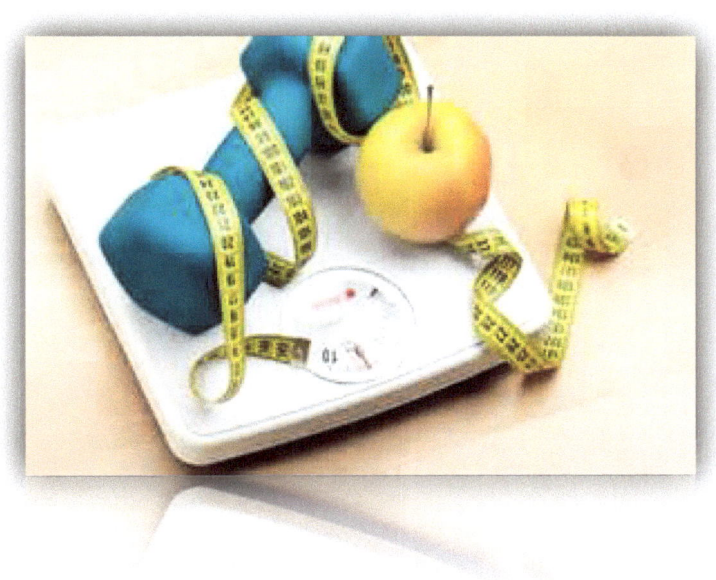

WEIGHT LOSS, NO GAIN!
RATHER THAN WEIGHT GAIN DURING THE
HOLIDAYS. HIGHLY POSSIBLE!

Weight-loss experts know that many people give up on diets during the holidays. Many overweight people have trouble getting back on track after the New Year. These healthy eating tips can help you lose weight during the season.

Several studies have shown that overweight people gain more weight during the holidays than non-overweight people. In one study, Drs. Baker and Kirschenbaum also found that overweight participants in professional weight control programs gained 500% more weight during holiday weeks compared to non-holiday weeks (in Health Psychology, 1998, 17: 367-370). Yes, this is indeed fact. Pay attention to it. I do always and constantly remind myself...

This means that holidays, with the continuous celebrations and ever-present high-fat and calorie-dense foods, are risky times for those who seek weight loss.

However, research also shows that weight controllers can not only learn to manage the challenges of the holidays, they can master them. Research has pointed to a number of critical elements of effective weight control during such high risk occasions.

Consider taking the following steps if you want to join the ranks of those actually lose weight during the holidays.

Establish a solid foundation on high-risk days.

The foundation for effective weight management is activity. Almost every study on individuals who succeed in maintaining weight loss over time shows that frequent activity contributes substantially to success.

So, on days with celebrations planned, if you begin the day with a brisk walk or some other activity, you are much more likely stay focused on your goals and get your body activated. Your metabolic rate (the amount of energy your body needs at rest) can either work for you or against you. If you stay active every day, you'll keep your metabolic rate from becoming too efficient (needing fewer calories).

In addition, controlled eating, especially in the morning, will also help you stay focused; building a foundation of the kind of habits that you'll need throughout your life for successful weight control.

Consider having a relatively high-protein breakfast (like an egg white omelet or fat-free cheese melted on an English muffin) to keep your hunger relatively quiet prior to the party.

Plan ahead.

When you plan ahead, you can predict and control your world. For example, think about your next party:

- Who is going to be there?

- What kind of food will be served?

- When are you going to leave?

You can call your host and get a preview of the menu. You can make a list of what you will eat, with whom you will talk, and how you will stay focused on successful weight control even during the party. Controlling alcohol intake may be critical along those lines. How about considering a 2-drink limit? That leads to better restraint and better focus on the big picture of your life.

Avoid starvation before celebration. Starving before a big holiday meal or party can increase the chances of binge eating. Starving produces deprivation and strong biological drives to eat anything. An alternative approach would have you eating low-fat low-sugar foods throughout the day as usual, and making sure to eat some source protein immediately prior to the event (e.g., low-fat beef or turkey jerky; fat-free cheese or yogurt).

Study the food scene. After arriving at the celebration, you can quickly survey the available options. Perhaps you will notice fresh fruits or vegetables that will work for your eating plan. You might also discover that the main course will keep you on target (for example, a turkey dinner can work very well). This initial survey should enable you to avoid the incredibly calorie-dense, high-fat chips and dips, nuts, and appetizers.

Monitor the details of your eating and activities. The research on this point is especially clear. Those who write down virtually everything they eat and their activities are far more likely to lose weight during the holidays, and during non-holiday weeks, as well. If you use goals for your eating plan (like no more than 20 fat grams per day), then by self-monitoring your eating every day, you can bring those goals to life – and use them as motivators. Every time you eat something, you compare that food to the 20 fat gram goal and see if you are on course to beat the goal. In a similar way, if you use a pedometer to keep track of your steps, then by monitoring the number of steps taken each day, you will encourage yourself to reach your step goal (like 10,000 steps per day).

Refocus your holiday season. You can break the holiday tradition of focusing on special foods and parties. Why not focus on other people, special projects, helping others, and finding new ways to relax?

5 HOW TO STAY ACTIVE?

How to stay active AND exercise during the holidays you ask?

Hmmm…I have the easy answers. Read on!

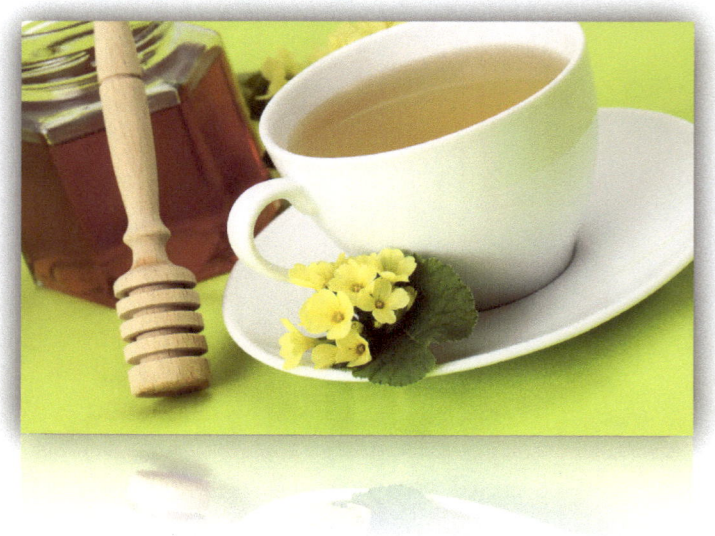

It's hard enough to exercise the rest of the year, but add holidays to the mix and many of us find exercise becomes less of a priority as to-do lists grow longer and longer.

The last thing you want is more stress and, for many of us, trying to keep to our usual workout program does just that.

At the same time, staying active in some way will give you energy, reduce stress and tension and, of course, help mitigate some of the extra calories you may be eating.

So, how do you find that balance? These quick tips will help you plan ahead, prepare yourself for any eventuality and provide workouts to help you stay active this holiday season.

Plan Ahead

If you're traveling, planning ahead can make all the difference. Take some time to figure out what your options are so you're ready for anything. Just a few ideas:

- Search for walking, running or park trails nearby

- Look up information about the hotel you're staying at and find out if they have an exercise room

- If you're staying with family, ask if they have any fitness equipment

- Talk to your family in advance and suggest taking a walk or doing something active together

- Plan simple workouts (see below) that don't require much space or equipment. If you're traveling or have visitors, you may be able to sneak in a workout in the basement without bothering anyone.

Try to plan your workout schedule beforehand. Even if you have to change it (which is likely when you're traveling), you've already made a commitment to exercise.

It's easier to stick with it when you have it planned than to squeeze it in later.

Get Prepared

If you're not sure about your schedule or whether you'll even have time to get in a workout, plan for the worst-case scenario.

That may be staying in grandma's basement with no equipment and only 10 or 15 minutes to your-self. Try these quick tips for squeezing in a workout even when you only have minutes to spare:

- Bring a workout plan with you. Plan a 10-minute routine you could do right in your bedroom. For example, you could choose 10 exercises and do each for 1 minute (squats, lunges, pushups, jumping jacks) or check out the holiday workouts below for other ideas.

- Bring resistance bands. They travel well and you can use them for quick strength exercises whenever you catch a few minutes.
- If guests are staying with you, move your equipment (weights or bands) into your bedroom so you can sneak in some exercise at night or in the morning.

- Wear your running or walking shoes as much as you can. You may find a 20-minute window when people are napping or before dinner for a quick walk or run.

You may even want to invite some family members for a walk. Sometimes there are others who'd love to work-out, but they're just waiting for someone else to step up first.

Use Every Opportunity

Planning and preparing are nice, but even the best-laid plans get derailed, especially during the holidays. If you find there's just no way to get in a workout, get creative and find ways to move your body any way you can:

- Walk as much as possible. Take extra laps at the mall, use the stairs, and volunteer to walk the dog.

- If you're hanging out with kids, set up a game of football, tag or hide and seek.

- Offer to help with the housework, shoveling snow or raking leaves.

- If everybody's sitting around watching football, get on the floor for some sit-ups or pushups. If that's too weird, try isometric exercises -- squeeze and hold the abs, the glutes or even press the hands together to engage the chest.

- If you don't have equipment, pick up some full water bottles or soup cans for quick lateral raises or overhead presses. Something is always better than nothing.

Holiday Workouts

If you need some workout ideas, these routines cover everything from cardio to circuit training to strength workouts with no equipment. Print them out and take them with you or just use them for inspiration in creating your own workouts.

The most important thing is to be realistic and go easy on your-self. You aren't always in charge of your schedule during the holidays so you can only do your best. Remind yourself that you can get back to your routine when you're backing home.

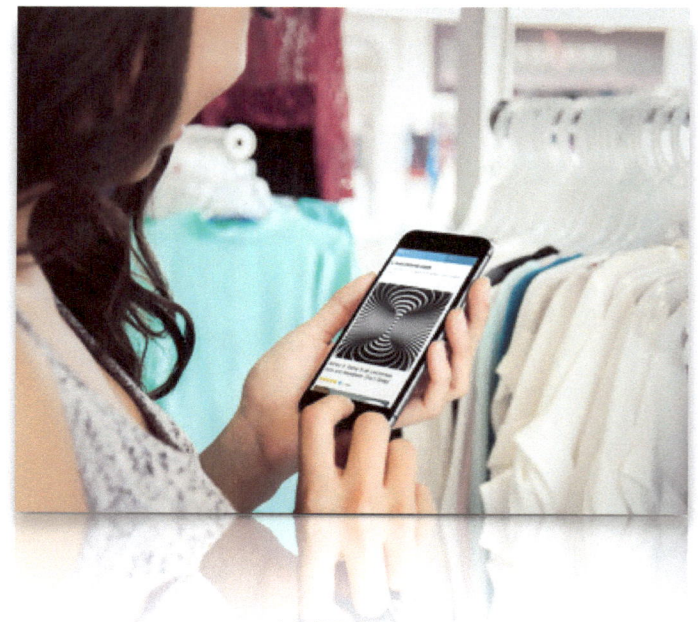

6 TIPS…

TIPS FOR USING FITNESS GADGETS…
…TO AVOID HOLIDA WEIGHT GAIN!

It's easy to gain weight during the holidays but tough to lose it. Over the years, that weight adds up. Here 10 fitness experts discuss how apps, wristbands, monitors and other technology can help you set and achieve fitness goals during the holiday season and far beyond.

During the holidays, you'll likely gain at least one pound, according to a study that appeared in the New England Journal of Medicine. While that doesn't sound like much, you probably won't lose that pound, either. As the years go by, those accumulated pounds become harder to shed. "This extra weight accumulates through the years and may be a major contributor to obesity later in life," the study says.

Not convinced? Just ask John Hennigan, also known as Johnny Nitro of World Wrestling Entertainment (WWE) fame. "It's way easier to keep weight off than to take it off," says the former wrestler, who has co-developed the Out of Your Mind Fitness training program. "Think about how much it takes to burn off a single Christmas cookie. Everyone who goes to the gym knows how much work they have put in, so why put it to waste in one weekend of gorging?"

Avoiding holiday weight gain, in theory, is as simple as setting realistic diet and exercise goals and sticking to them. But that's not so easy when, between Thanksgiving and New Year's Day, you're perpetually teased by ham, turkey, mashed potatoes, stuffing, pumpkin pie, eggnog, wine, cookies, cakes, you name it.

Fortunately, there's no shortage of affordable consumer tech to help: Activity trackers such as Fit bit; mobile apps for counting calories, such as My Fitness Pal; Nintendo Wii fitness games; heart-rate monitors, and Wi-Fi-enabled bathroom scales, such as the Within Smart Body Analyzer, which sync your weight and other stats with diet and fitness apps.

To help you stay fit during the holidays, we asked 10 tech-savvy health and fitness experts about the technology they use for diet and exercise as well as their strategies for staying fit.

Choose tech that best matches your goals. "For technology to be effective, you need to start with strong, well-thought-out goals and determine your tactics to achieve them," says Michael Rucker, director of digital products at Club One fitness centers in the San Francisco Bay Area. "This might seem fairly straightforward, but I can't tell you how many indoor cyclists I've seen [who've] purchase a popular accelerometer, like a Fit bit or Jawbone, and then quickly become frustrated because, given their fitness affinity, they'd have been better off with a heart-rate monitor."

Fitness consultant and personal trainer Amie Hoff of FitKit.com recommends that you first decide which activity you like doing and want to track. Also, determine your top health priority, whether it's elevating your heart rate, losing weight or toning your body. Finally, take into account where you would want to wear a device: Wrist, belt or chest.

Do your homework. Read reviews of activity trackers, heart-rate monitors and other gear before you buy, says Ted Vickey, senior consultant for technology at the American Council on Exercise. In addition to checking out professional reviews on tech sites, look at user reviews on Amazon.com, REI.com and other e-commerce sites.

Look for ease of use. We all have enough excuses not to be physically active, Vickey says. An activity tracker or other tech device that's not easy to use gives us yet another reason to be inactive.

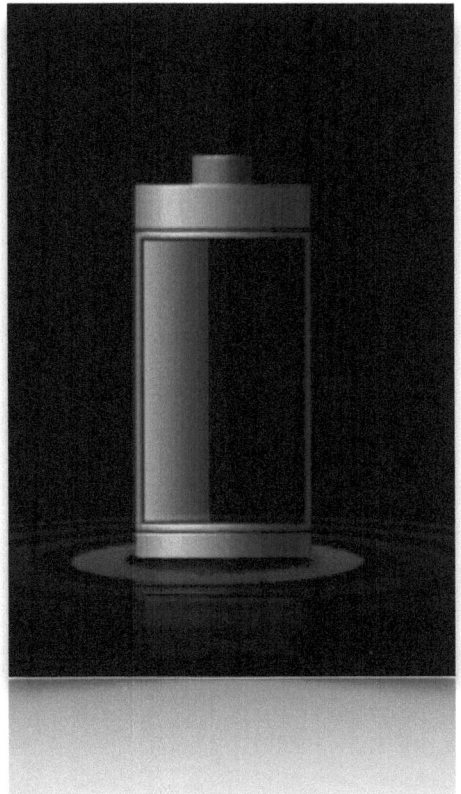

Check the retailer's return policy. If you're planning on wearing, say, a Nike+ Fuel Band every day, you should make sure you're going to love it. But you might not know how you feel about the device for a few weeks, maybe even a month. That's why it pays to check return policies. For example, REI lets you return a product up to one year after purchase (except for items purchased from REI's online outlet store). Best Buy offers 45-day returns for Elite Plus members, but only 15 days for everyone else.

Lose things easily? Wear an activity tracker on your wrist. Many people like the Fit bit one tracker ($100). But the device, which clips to a belt or bra or slips into a pocket, can also end up in the washing machine which can destroy it. Or you may lose it. (That said, when a friend lost his Fitbit, someone found it and notified the device maker, which in turn located the owner and arranged to have his Fitbit sent back to him.) If either of those scenarios seem likely, you'd be better off with an activity tracker worn on your wrist. These include the Fit bit Flex ($100), Fit bit Force ($130), Jawbone UP ($130), or Nike+ Fuel Band SE ($150).

Don't get too dazzled by tech. "Most people go for top-of-the-line devices with lots of bells and whistles, only to get overwhelmed, not know how to set it up or understand how to read the results. And then they never use it," Hoff says. "I suggest people go for the basic device that meets their needs or one you can grow into. I also recommend borrowing a friend's device and trying it for a day or two."

Don't let tech get you into a rut. "Frequently, I see boring fitness routines caused by reliance on technology," says Doug Piller, owner and lead trainer at Cross Fit Go Time in San Diego. For example, you may walk the same 10,000 steps every day because your Fitbit tracks those steps. "But you shouldn't get complacent in your fitness routine. I recommend switching up your routine constantly, rotating between different methods of strength-training and cardio. Get creative. Try a different way of burning calories: Swimming, hiking with your pet, CrossFit, sprint intervals, dancing with your favorite Wii game or doing hot yoga."

Don't let your device distract you. "Your smartphone or tablet can be a wealth of fitness information while you're at the gym," says former wrestler Hennigan. "But it can also be distracting. I regularly see people swiping touchscreens, starting new playlists and answering texts mid-workout.

Hennigan does use his smartphone to play music while working out, but he usually puts it in airplane mode so he doesn't get any texts, tweets, or calls while he's training. "I often use my phone as an oversized timer," he adds. "This works well for fight training to simulate rounds, to time sections of your workout like dynamic warm-ups and stretching, or isometric exercises."

Get social. Many activity trackers and diet/exercise apps include a social media component. For example, Fitbit's website and mobile apps lets you see how many steps your other Fitbit-owning friends have walked in a given week (provided they agree to share their data with you). Sharing your stats can make you more competitive as well as keep you accountable.

Also, the social media connect "creates a community," Hoff says. "People know there are others out there struggling just like them. They have a place to share their struggles and triumphs. Social media encourages success, offers support, and it's a great place to find tips, tricks and tools that others have found."

Get rewarded. Some diet and fitness apps connect with fitness trackers and help you earn rewards for your activities. Some examples include Earned It, for perks and charitable donations; Fit Cause, which connects with Nike + Fuel Bands and lets you help charities through fitness, and Gym-Pact, an Android and iOS apps that earn you money for exercising but costs you money if you slack off.

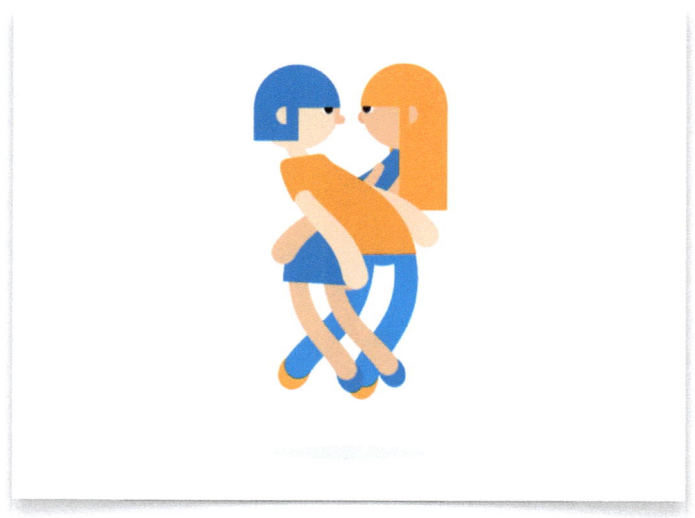

7 CONCLUSION

In conclusion, the final component to this weight control

plan is simply having a calendar to track your progress.

However, you must have your own separate calendar because you and your training partner will produce different results. The benefit of having a calendar is that you can track your progress over days, weeks and months.

Firstly, mark down the "work out days" that best suits your time schedule, as it only needs to be done 3 days a week. Generally if there are any dates you miss, it will motivate you to make up it.

Finally, simply write down your weight for the week to see how your weight loss progress has been.

*Balance it out...*Keep in mind that you're eating plan and calendar must be done **DAILY** while your workouts should be on the same days for every week to keep it consistent. As you can see a weight control plan is much easier than most people think. The key to weight loss is just consistency and commitment to this simple, yet effective weight control plan. All the three components are important and they can all work around any busy life schedule.

I wish all of **YOU** Angels the best holdalls possible. Stay warm, safe, eat **RIGHT** and **BALANCED**. Eat healthy. Get good night's rest all the time. This a key component as you now know as well…

May your **BEFORE**, **DURING** and **AFTER** holidays' days be filled with   lots of warmth, love and lots of happy returns. Don't mess with the weight thing again!

Bless You!

Regards,

Lisa Kristinardottir

xoxo kisses & hugs

Winter Holidays 2014-2015

During and Beyond!

Happy Times for YOU and YOURS!

LISASGAMEAPPS.COM | LISASLOCATOR.COM

www.ingramcontent.com/pod-product-compliance
Lightning Source LLC
Chambersburg PA
CBHW050823290526
45792CB00001B/237